Rock Bottom

Don't make your home there

By Dave Puddle

I dedicate this book to Jacky, Natalie, Nadine, Katrina, and Leander who stood with me when I was at Rock Bottom

Introduction

This will not be a long read because when I was at rock bottom the idea of reading was not top of my list. I had been an avid reader but found reading very difficult at that time in my life. I just couldn't concentrate.

Once upon a time, there was an elderly gentleman who kept a lovely white canary in a very clean cage in his living room and the canary would often sing throughout the day. On one particular day, the gentleman decided to clean his carpet and so got out the hoover and started to clean the living room. As he was near the cage he saw there were quite a few bits on the floor of the cage and so he decided to quickly hoover those bits up. As he placed the hoover extension in the cage there was a knock at the door and for a split second he turned around and in that very moment the hoover sucked up the beautiful white canary. Down it shot into the dirt and filth of the hoover bag. When the gentleman realised what he had done he was horrified and immediately switched off the hoover. He took the hoover bag out and searched until he found his lovely white canary which was now rather black and dirty. He cleaned the canary up as best as he could and placed it back in its cage. Sadly, from that day on the canary never sang again. The effect of being sucked up into the hoover bag had caused the canary to lose its song. Like that canary, we can be sucked up into the hoover of life, which contains all the filth and horribleness of life and we also can lose our song and get to a place in our lives where we are at rock bottom. It happened to me and I guess because you are reading this book it has happened to you or someone very close to you.

My sole purpose in writing this book is to encourage you that, yes, you may be at rock bottom but that is not a place where you have to stay. You can begin to climb up. It won't be easy but you can do it.

So come and share my journey, and as you read this I hope you will begin your journey of recovery. The address where your journey commences is called Rock Bottom, School of Life, Somewhere in the universe. It is not a physical location and yet it is a very real place, right at the forefront of your mind. A place you would not deliberately set out to find or dwell at, but nevertheless, it is the place where you now find yourself living. A place you would not even wish your worst enemy to be living at. So together let's decide that this is not a place either of us wishes to make as our permanent home.

And so let the journey begin.

Chapter 1 How did I get to this place known as Rock Bottom?

For about thirty years I had been a church minister. For the outsider looking in it might have appeared that I had gained a measure of success. Over that thirty year period, I had married people, buried people, counseled people. Helped the person who was suicidal to not take his own life. The couple who had their house repossessed I was able to sort it so that they could once again take ownership of the same house. Stood with the person who was standing in the dock in the high court, helped those who were threatened with eviction from their property and those who had got themselves into financial difficulty. Yes, my job had indeed been very varied, but here I was in my mid-fifties no longer myself. My wife and family had known for some time that I was ill but as usual, being a man that was not something I wanted to admit to. I thought give it a week or so and I would be better. However, one week turned into two, and then that turned into a month and I was getting progressively worse until the time came when I had to admit that I was ill. I would only go and see my doctor if my wife came with me.
There in the doctor's surgery what should have been a routine five minute appointment turned into nearly an hour long appointment with me being a total

blubbering wreck. I only said to the GP 'I feel so low' and with that flood loads of tears came streaming out. Over the course of the next fifty minutes or so I had to admit to just how bad things were, that on more than one occasion I had contemplated suicide and that I had kept all this stuff from my wife and family.

So I was diagnosed with severe depression, total body exhaustion, and having a nervous breakdown. All saying the same thing, that I was unwell. I felt at rock bottom and now I had a diagnosis to go along with where I found myself. Then started the medication, weekly trips to the GP, appointments to see the psychiatrist, and a counselor. I was in a real mess.

The medication took me out of myself and so I began to cope better but I was still at rock bottom.
One thing I learnt from this is that there is very little point in trying to understand how you arrived at rock bottom because that does not make one iota of difference. You are already in that place. Analysing how you got there does not stop you from being in that place. It is a bit like going on a car journey and when going down the road you suddenly hear one of your tyres making a strange noise and you just know you have to pull over to the side because you have developed a puncture. When that happens, you get

on the phone to the breakdown team and they send someone to fix your car and get you moving again. What you don't do is start examining the tyre to see what has caused the puncture. You don't start walking back up the road trying to find where that object might have come from. In a nutshell, you don't focus on the past you focus on the future, getting the tyre repaired and continuing on your journey.

It is the same when you find yourself at rock bottom. You cannot focus on the past and how you got there, you must focus on the future and how you are going to move on from this place.

When you walk through a graveyard and take the time to read the words on the gravestone there is always one character you see no matter how long or how short the writing is. That character is -. You find it between the day they were born and the day that person died. E.g. 1934 – 2019, and that hyphen represents all that individual's life; the highs and the lows, the good and the bad, the successes and the failures. One day, if we have a gravestone or a plaque with our name on then we too will have a hyphen, and contained within that hyphen, will be the fact that at a particular point of time in our life we were at a place called rock bottom.

For me arriving at rock bottom didn't happen that at

one point in my life everything was fine and following a bad night's sleep I woke up at rock bottom. No, it was a gradual process. At the time I was totally unaware of what was going on but now looking back I can see that there were signs that I was heading for rock bottom. However, as I have said there is no point in looking back. We must keep looking forward.

Being at rock bottom does not mean that we are worthless or useless, it just means that at this particular time in our life we are in a very difficult place. Unless you have been in that place no one knows what it is like. They can only imagine and imagining is nowhere near the same as being in that place. I would tell myself to pull yourself together and yet I couldn't. I would tell myself to get a grip and yet I couldn't. I would tell myself to stop crying and yet I couldn't. I would tell myself I am not in this place but I was. I had to admit I was at rock bottom.

There is not a one size fits all for the journey to the place of rock bottom, there are many roads that can lead you to rock bottom. However, there is a very real place called rock bottom and if you find yourself there you need to realise you are not the only one there. There could be thousands of people who are at rock bottom at exactly the same time you find yourself there, yet being at rock bottom can be the loneliest place on planet earth. Yes rock bottom may exist in our minds but it is played out in life and life can be very lonely. You can be surrounded by a loving family, have great friends, be part of the in crowd and yet you can be incredibly lonely. Rock bottom is not the place where we want to make our home.

For the outsider looking in they probably wonder how you can even imagine you are at rock bottom when there are people much worse off than yourself. That may very well be true but it does not distract from how you feel, and if you believe you are at rock bottom then you probably are.

For me, when I first reached rock bottom, it felt very much that rock bottom was the place where I was going to spend the rest of my life. People kept saying things would get better but I just didn't believe them. All I could see was darkness, misery, and pain. It was just so bleak.

I felt I was at the bottom of a very big hole feeling so small and when looking up all I could see were people getting on with their lives. I felt so small, so insignificant, with no way out. There were no ladders to help me climb the walls, there were no steps embedded in the walls to get a foothold. The walls were just straight and vertical with not a mark on them. I felt truly trapped.

Chapter 2 Living through rock bottom.

Everything in Rock Bottom appears heavy and hard. It is a very dark, cold, and lonely place.

Despite being on the medication at that time it certainly didn't feel like it was helping. There was no magical instant cure for where I found myself at. Numerous mornings I would not want to get out of bed but from somewhere deep within I made myself get up. It might have been a loving family member encouraging me to get dressed, or the fact that I had to get dressed to show my downs syndrome/autistic daughter that daddy was ok.

Getting dressed was hard enough and then on top of that, I had to get a wash. I was quite happy with greasy hair, an unshaven face. Left to my own devices I would probably have been at rock bottom longer.

What once was easy and routine now became difficult and daunting. We had had many family holidays, some in this country and some abroad. I vividly remember being at rock bottom and having to navigate to go to an airport, to get on an airplane, to go on a holiday that had been booked a number of months before. All those people in the airport caused me so much anxiety it was unreal. Previously I had been the one in charge of the tickets and passports but this time no way – too much pressure I just could not cope with it. Thankfully my family was great and looked after me.

How you see yourself and how others see you are probably miles apart. I saw myself as a useless nobody who was better off dead and that my family would be much better off without me. Yet they saw me as a loving husband, father who contributed to the wellbeing of family life.

At rock bottom not only do you not think straight, but you also do not see things clearly either. Everything you look at can be viewed through a lens of dirty corrupt glasses. You feel unlovable and yet there are those who love you. You feel you are of no value and yet there are those who say you bring value to their life. It really is a topsy turvy place to try and navigate through, so much harder because being in that place means that we are no longer thinking clearly, logically, or correctly.

We must learn to listen to what those who love us are truly saying to us. There is so much noise that wants to control our brains and we need to make sure to tune out all the bad stuff and allow the good stuff in. At times we need to hear things from our family which we would rather not hear. All we want is to be left alone, for that is how we feel when we are at rock bottom. Somehow we must fight to overcome the self-isolation we so crave. Just to be left alone to sit in our dark cave is so appealing and yet it is also so wrong. When we are sat in our cave it is so dark and lonely and before we know it our mind begins to play tricks with us. Words just appear out of nowhere, and yes ninety-nine percent of the time those words are truly negative words. Those negative words become audible negative words right into the center of our minds when we are all alone in our cave at rock bottom. Those words seek to tell us who we are, what we should do and no matter how hard you try to tune those words out, they constantly seem to bombard you from every direction. I found there was only one way I could get those negative words to be silent and that was to somehow find a way to hear different words. Those words were not necessarily positive words but words that did not immediately impact my mental well-being. It was a case of thinking about other subjects, whether it be sport, films or even the weather. Anything just to break the cycle of negativity about myself that I was constantly hearing. The cycle needed to be broken and for me it was not sorted after one attempt, I had to keep doing it as often as I needed to. Those words and thoughts do not just come once a day, but many times throughout the day. I finally came to a place where I knew what I needed to do, and then I had to find the inner strength to actually do what was required. Never easy when you are at the place I call rock bottom.

Life was a constant battle and uphill struggle but, without realising it, I was beginning to move away from rock bottom.

Once rock bottom has got its teeth into you it does not want to let you go. It wants to keep you there for the rest of your life. The bombardment of negative words, the inability to see any future for yourself is all designed to keep you within its dark clutches. There is a saying which says, 'there is always light at the end of the tunnel,' but I have to confess that for a considerable length of time I could see no light at the end of the tunnel I was encapsulated within. Above me, below me, to the sides of me, as far as I could see forward and backward there was only thick black darkness. All it would take would be for the light of a small lit match to dispel the darkness, but there was no match. If only a single star would shine, but there was no star. Just a blanket of darkness. It truly was a horrible place.

In the midst of these dark days, I would occasionally have a good day. What did that mean? Well things did not appear so dark and without hope, but sadly those moments didn't last, they were soon overcome by the forces of darkness.

Chapter 3 Make a couple of victories

If possible set yourself at least a couple of achievable goals each day. They do not have to be hard but, depending on how you are feeling, not too easy.

The first goal I set myself each day was simply to get out of bed. When everything is fine getting out of bed is no problem, even if you have a long lay in, but in Rock Bottom, it can be one of the hardest things to do. Your mind and body are yelling at you to stay in bed, keep the covers up to your neck, keep your eyes shut, however, we have to get up otherwise another victory goes to remaining at rock bottom. We might require a goal in order to get up. It may be to take the children to school, to hoover the living room, or something entirely different, but a goal is a tool to help you accomplish something for that day.

The second goal I set myself was to go out for a walk each day. At rock bottom, the last thing you want to do is to go outside the four walls of your home, come castle. Staying within the four walls keeps us in control of who, if anybody, we see. Being in the castle feels the safest place to be. It becomes a real battle to go out but it is a victory we need to chalk up. It might be a case of just going out for a five minute walk after dark so no one can see you or bump into you for a quick chat. At times when I was out for a walk and would see someone I knew coming towards me, I would get my mobile phone and pretend to be in deep conversation, therefore all I had to do was just nod. I always allowed some distance to be in place before I put my phone back into my pocket after the conversation with my imaginary friend. Even walking five minutes a day will be of help to you. Gradually build it up to somewhere between 30 minutes and one hour. By doing this, over time you will begin to see an improvement in how you feel. It will not only help with your mental health but also with your physical health as well. You will get a little fitter and maybe lose some weight if you have been comfort eating during your time at rock bottom.

Chapter 4 The power of words

Words are incredibly powerful. What you say both outwardly and inwardly can have a profound impact on you. Have you ever convinced yourself that you were unwell by keep saying, 'I don't feel well.' Of course, when we think we are ill and keep getting a headache we automatically focus on the worst case scenario, I think I may have a brain tumour. Never once does it occur to us that it may be because we are not getting enough sleep, or the room is too stuffy, or even you may have been drinking too much coffee. More often than not sentences are either positive or negative. These sentences are made up of words. Think about how the following two short sentences make you feel.

I love you. I hate you.

One makes you feel good about yourself and the other makes you feel bad about yourself. When we hear those words it conjures up images in our mind of just what those words are saying to us.

It is important that when we are at rock bottom that we hear positive words, both audible and also those in our minds. Everything within us is screaming negativity but we need to find the strength to say, that is not the whole picture. There is someone out there who loves me. There is someone out there who values me. If you can put a name to that someone then try and speak it out loud, e.g. Jacky loves me. My work colleagues value me. Try doing this, you have nothing to lose and everything to gain.

Two small words are 'can' and 'will.' I can get out of bed. I will get out of bed. Small words yet different words. 'I can' implies that if I want to I am able to do whatever it is. 'I will' implies that I will do whatever it is. So when you are laid in bed think, I will get up. By saying this it will help you to get out of bed. I will go for a walk. It is basically you telling your body what you are going to be doing, and not allowing your body to tell you what it wants to be doing. Try making that small change in a number of areas where you are currently struggling and see if it makes a difference. It is amazing how even a very small change can have quite a profound impact upon your life when you are at rock bottom.

Chapter 5 Meditate

When you are at rock bottom you long to be somewhere else, this can be achieved through meditation. It took me quite a number of attempts before I was able to go to that place in my mind, but I persevered and succeeded. I was so glad I did because of the benefit it brought into my daily living. There is nothing mystical about meditating the way that I did it. The idea was to think of a place where I would be happy, visualise it, and believe you are at that place. This is what I did. I would go to my room where it was quiet. Sit in a comfortable chair and close my eyes. Then I would think that I was sitting on a sun drenched tropical white sandy beach with a large coconut tree overhanging to the left and the sun beaming down. There would be greenery all around this lovely little sandy cove and I was the only one on the beach. I would sit relaxing and watch the turquoise coloured waves come in and gently break on the beach. At times I would even be able to hear the sound of the waves. I would often spend many minutes in this place for it was a place of calm and beauty. Yes, it was all in my mind but at the time it felt a very real place. It was a great way to escape from being at rock bottom.

You need to find a place where you feel relaxed and happy and then meditate to be at that place. It might be helpful to have some quiet relaxing music in the background as you close your eyes and gently begin to relax and think of such a place.

If you don't achieve this on your first number of attempts, keep at it because you will get there. Just relax and try to let everything go from your mind, think about that happy and relaxing place. Soon you will be there.

Chapter 6 What do you see

Being at rock bottom all I could see was doom, gloom, and pain. I saw no future and the present was horrible. I could not even focus on the day ahead, let alone six months or a year.

When we are at rock bottom we can only see the present, not the future. It is as if, with our eyes, we can only ever see our immediate surroundings. We need to hold on to the fact that one day we will once again fly like an eagle and see far into the distance. The higher the eagle flies, the further the eagle can see.

Why not pretend that today you are an eagle, look into the distance at where you want to be in six months or a year's time. Write it down and hold on to that dream. It might be that you see yourself no longer at rock bottom and once again enjoying life. It might be that in a year's time you can see yourself once again going on holiday. Hold on to it and if necessary read it each day to remind yourself that, no matter how you are feeling today, you still do have a future.

Try asking a family member to write down how they imagine you to be in six months or a year's time. This is not to put any pressure on you but to show you that others believe you are going to get better, and they also believe that you are going to leave rock bottom. It is amazing how much faith others have that you will indeed get better.

I hope you have found this book helpful.

If you wish to contact me please feel free

davegpcwork@outlook.com

www.ingramcontent.com/pod-product-compliance
Lightning Source LLC
Chambersburg PA
CBHW031512210526
45463CB00008B/3208